Cancer Control
Knowledge into Action
WHO Guide for Effective Programmes

D1303824

Planning

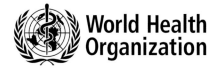

World Health Organization

WHO Library Cataloguing-in-Publication Data

Planning.
(Cancer control : knowledge into action : WHO guide for effective programmes ; module 1.)
1.Neoplasms – prevention and control. 2.Health planning. 3.National health programs – organization and administration. 4.Health policy. 5.Guidelines. I.World Health Organization. II.Series.
ISBN 92 4 154699 9   (NLM classification: QZ 200)

The Cancer Control Planning module was produced under the overall direction of Catherine Le Galès-Camus (Assistant Director-General, Noncommunicable Diseases and Mental Health), Robert Beaglehole (Director, Chronic Diseases and Health Promotion) and Serge Resnikoff (Coordinator, Chronic Diseases Prevention and Management).

Cecilia Sepúlveda, coordinator of the overall publication, coordinated this module and provided extensive editorial input.

Inés Salas acted as adviser and provided valuable technical guidance. Editorial support was provided by Anthony Miller (scientific editor) and Angela Haden (technical writer and editor). Proofreading was done by Ann Morgan.

The production of the module was coordinated by Maria Villanueva.

Core contributions for the module were received from the following experts:

Robert Burton, National Cancer Control Initiative, Australia
Margaret Fitch, International Society of Nurses in Cancer Care and Canada, Canada
Leslie S. Given, Centers for Disease Control and Prevention, USA
Jon F. Kerner, National Cancer Institute, USA
Mónica Ortegón, WHO, Switzerland
Paula Pisani, International Agency for Research on Cancer, France
Inés Salas, University of Santiago, Chile
Cecilia Sepúlveda, WHO, Switzerland

Other people also contributed by providing country examples through telephone interviews and personal communication for this module and for the web site:

Anderson S. Doh, Faculty of Medicine and Biomedical Sciences, Cameroon
Nguyen Ba Duc, National Cancer Hospital, Viet Nam
Miklós Kásler, National Institute of Oncology, Hungary
Lingzhi Kong, Ministry of Health, China
M. Krishnan Nair, Regional Cancer Centre, India
Reto Obrist, Oncosuisse, Switzerland
Azhar M. Qureshi, Al-Ihsan Hospital, Pakistan
K. Raamamoorthy, Ministry of Health and Family Welfare, India
Dolores Salas Trejo, Department of Health, Regional Government of Valencia, Spain
Simon Sutcliffe, British Columbia Cancer Agency, Canada
Colin Tukuitonga, WHO, Switzerland
Marjan van Waardenberg, Ministry of Health, New Zealand

Valuable input, help and advice were received from a number of people in WHO headquarters throughout the production of the module: Caroline Allsopp, David Bramley, Robert Constandse, Raphaël Crettaz, JoAnne Epping-Jordan, Maryvonne Grisetti, Jane McElligott and Alexandra Touchaud. Cancer experts worldwide, as well as technical staff in headquarters and in regional and country offices, also provided valuable input by making contributions and reviewing the module, and are listed in the Acknowledgements.

Design and layout: L'IV Com Sàrl, Morges, Switzerland.

Printed in Switzerland

More information about this publication can be obtained from:
Department of Chronic Diseases and Health Promotion
World Health Organization
CH-1211 Geneva 27
Switzerland

The production of this publication was made possible through the generous financial support of the National Cancer Institute (NCI), USA. We would also like to thank the National Cancer Institute of France (INCa), the Public Health Agency of Canada (PHAC), the International Atomic Energy Agency (IAEA), and the International Union Against Cancer (UICC) for their financial support.

Introduction to the
Cancer Control Series

Cancer is to a large extent avoidable. Many cancers can be prevented. Others can be detected early in their development, treated and cured. Even with late stage cancer, the pain can be reduced, the progression of the cancer slowed, and patients and their families helped to cope.

Cancer is a leading cause of death globally. The World Health Organization estimates that 7.6 million people died of cancer in 2005 and 84 million people will die in the next 10 years if action is not taken. More than 70% of all cancer deaths occur in low- and middle-income countries, where resources available for prevention, diagnosis and treatment of cancer are limited or nonexistent.

But because of the wealth of available knowledge, all countries can, at some useful level, implement the four basic components of cancer control – *prevention, early detection, diagnosis and treatment, and palliative care* – and thus avoid and cure many cancers, as well as palliating the suffering.

Cancer control: knowledge into action, WHO guide for effective programmes is a series of six modules that provides practical advice for programme managers and policy-makers on how to advocate, plan and implement effective cancer control programmes, particularly in low- and middle-income countries.

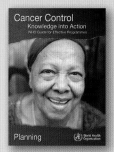

PLANNING
A practical guide for programme managers on how to plan overall cancer control effectively, according to available resources and integrating cancer control with programmes for other chronic diseases and related problems.

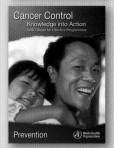

PREVENTION
A practical guide for programme managers on how to implement effective cancer prevention by controlling major avoidable cancer risk factors.

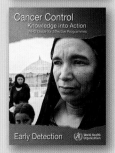

EARLY DETECTION
A practical guide for programme managers on how to implement effective early detection of major types of cancer that are amenable to early diagnosis and screening.

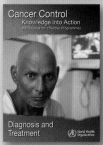

DIAGNOSIS AND TREATMENT
A practical guide for programme managers on how to implement effective cancer diagnosis and treatment, particularly linked to early detection programmes or curable cancers.

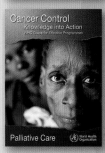

PALLIATIVE CARE
A practical guide for programme managers on how to implement effective palliative care for cancer, with a particular focus on community-based care.

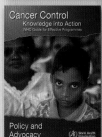

POLICY AND ADVOCACY
A practical guide for medium level decision-makers and programme managers on how to advocate for policy development and effective programme implementation for cancer control.

The WHO guide is a response to the World Health Assembly resolution on cancer prevention and control (WHA58.22), adopted in May 2005, which calls on Member States to intensify action against cancer by developing and reinforcing cancer control programmes. It builds on *National cancer control programmes: policies and managerial guidelines* and *Preventing chronic diseases: a vital investment*, as well as on the various WHO policies that have influenced efforts to control cancer.

Cancer control aims to reduce the incidence, morbidity and mortality of cancer and to improve the quality of life of cancer patients in a defined population, through the systematic implementation of evidence-based interventions for prevention, early detection, diagnosis, treatment, and palliative care. Comprehensive cancer control addresses the whole population, while seeking to respond to the needs of the different subgroups at risk.

COMPONENTS OF CANCER CONTROL

Prevention of cancer, especially when integrated with the prevention of chronic diseases and other related issues (such as reproductive health, hepatitis B immunization, HIV/AIDS, occupational and environmental health), offers the greatest public health potential and the most cost-effective long-term method of cancer control. We now have sufficient knowledge to prevent around 40% of all cancers. Most cancers are linked to tobacco use, unhealthy diet, or infectious agents (see Prevention module).

Early detection detects (or diagnoses) the disease at an early stage, when it has a high potential for cure (e.g. cervical or breast cancer). Interventions are available which permit the early detection and effective treatment of around one third of cases (see Early Detection module).

There are two strategies for early detection:
- *early diagnosis*, often involving the patient's awareness of early signs and symptoms, leading to a consultation with a health provider – who then promptly refers the patient for confirmation of diagnosis and treatment;

- *national or regional screening* of asymptomatic and apparently healthy individuals to detect pre-cancerous lesions or an early stage of cancer, and to arrange referral for diagnosis and treatment.

Treatment aims to cure disease, prolong life, and improve the quality of remaining life after the diagnosis of cancer is confirmed by the appropriate available procedures. The most effective and efficient treatment is linked to early detection programmes and follows evidence-based standards of care. Patients can benefit either by cure or by prolonged life, in cases of cancers that although disseminated are highly responsive to treatment, including acute leukaemia and lymphoma. This component also addresses rehabilitation aimed at improving the quality of life of patients with impairments due to cancer (see Diagnosis and Treatment module).

Palliative care meets the needs of all patients requiring relief from symptoms and of psychosocial and supportive care, particularly those with advanced stages who have a very low chance of being cured or who are facing the terminal phase of the disease. Cancer and its management have emotional, spiritual, social and economic consequences for patients and their family members. For them, palliative care services addressing their needs from the time of diagnosis can influence their quality of life and their ability to cope effectively (see Palliative Care module).

Despite cancer being a global public health problem, many governments have not yet included cancer control in their health agendas. There are competing health problems, and interventions may be chosen in response to the demands of interest groups, rather than in response to population needs or on the basis of cost-effectiveness and affordability.

Low-income and disadvantaged groups are generally more exposed to avoidable cancer risk factors, such as environmental carcinogens, tobacco use, alcohol abuse and infectious agents. These groups have less political influence, less access to health services, and lack education that can empower them to make decisions to protect and improve their own health.

BASIC PRINCIPLES OF CANCER CONTROL

- **Leadership** to create clarity and unity of purpose, and to encourage team building, broad participation, ownership of the process, continuous learning and mutual recognition of efforts made.

- **Involvement of stakeholders** of all related sectors, and at all levels of the decision-making process, to enable active participation and commitment of key players for the benefit of the programme.

- **Creation of partnerships** to enhance effectiveness through mutually beneficial relationships, and build upon trust and complementary capacities of partners from different disciplines and sectors.

- **Responding to the needs of people** at risk of developing cancer or already presenting with the disease, in order to meet their physical, psychosocial and spiritual needs across the full continuum of care.

- **Decision-making** based on evidence, social values and efficient and cost-effective use of resources that benefit the target population in a sustainable and equitable way.

- **Application of a systemic approach** by implementing a comprehensive programme with interrelated key components sharing the same goals and integrated with other related programmes and to the health system.

- **Seeking continuous improvement,** innovation and creativity to maximize performance and to address social and cultural diversity, as well as the needs and challenges presented by a changing environment.

- **Adoption of a stepwise approach** to planning and implementing interventions, based on local considerations and needs. (see next page for WHO stepwise framework for chronic diseases prevention and control, as applied to cancer control).

WHO stepwise framework

1

PLANNING STEP 1
Where are we now?

Investigate the present state of the cancer problem, and cancer control services or programmes.

2

PLANNING STEP 2
Where do we want to be?

Formulate and adopt policy. This includes defining the target population, setting goals and objectives, and deciding on priority interventions across the cancer continuum.

3

PLANNING STEP 3
How do we get there?

Identify the steps needed to implement the policy.

The planning phase is followed by the policy implementation phase.

Implementation step 1
CORE

Implement interventions in the policy that are feasible now, with existing resources.

Implementation step 2
EXPANDED

Implement interventions in the policy that are feasible in the medium term, with a realistically projected increase in, or reallocation of, resources.

Implementation step 3
DESIRABLE

Implement interventions in the policy that are beyond the reach of current resources, if and when such resources become available.

PLANNING MODULE CONTENTS

KEY MESSAGES

Planning involves:

" An honest understanding of an organization's history. A systematic examination of an organization's environment. The rigorous assessment of an organization's mission. Clear vision of organizational goals. A mapping process presenting ways of reaching those goals. An inclusive, collaborative process for gathering information, ideas, opinions and intuitions on which goals and decisions are based. A realization that planning never stops. "

Source: Taylor E. *Trick or treat (or why plan?)*
(http://www.nea.gov/resources/Lessons/TAYLOR.HTML, accessed 18 May 2006).

Cancer control planning is necessary in any resource setting in order to respond to the cancer needs in populations by preventing cancer, detecting it early, curing it and caring for people affected by it. This module addresses some basic aspects of planning, and discusses how to determine whether a plan is needed and, if so, how to draw up a strategic plan.

key definitions

What is a plan?

- ▣ A plan is a set of intended actions that are expected to achieve a specified goal within a certain time frame.
- ▣ "A good plan is like a road map: it shows the final destination and usually the best way to get there."

Judd HS. H. Stanley Judd Quotes (http://en.thinkexist.com/quotes/h._stanley_judd/ accessed 18 May 2006).

The key messages for people involved in cancer control planning and implementation are as follows:

☐ An integrated, comprehensive cancer control strategy allows for a more balanced, efficient and equitable use of limited resources.

☐ In order to plan cancer control wisely, it is necessary to understand the context, appreciate past experiences, and be ready to learn continuously.

☐ A cancer control plan that is goal-oriented, people-centred, realistic and carefully prepared through a participatory process is more likely to move into effective implementation.

☐ In lower-resource settings, a plan that considers the gradual implementation of a few, affordable, cost-effective and priority interventions will have a better chance of moving into effective action.

This module is complemented by various practical tools accessible through the WHO cancer web site
http://www.who.int/cancer

WWW

What is a programme?

A programme is the organized and systematic implementation of the actions described in the plan, according to a defined time frame and using defined resources (human, physical and financial).

What is a planning process?

Planning is a formalized procedure, in the form of an integrated system of decisions, to produce an articulated result. Thinking about, and attempting to control, the future are important components of planning (Mintzberg, 1994).

3

PRE-PLANNING

With careful planning, a substantial degree of cancer control can be achieved, even where resources are limited. Without careful planning, there is a risk that the resources available for cancer control will be used inefficiently, and that the benefits to the population that should flow from these resources will not be realized.

> Several countries have introduced national cancer plans that provide good models of how to proceed, see http://www.who.int/cancer for examples.
>
> WWW

IS A NEW CANCER CONTROL PLAN NEEDED?

There is no country in the world where cancer does not occur. Even in low-resource countries, some level of cancer control activity is going on. Effective cancer control plans are thus needed everywhere. Reasons for initiating a cancer control planning process, or for updating an existing plan might be:

- there is no previously written cancer control plan in the country or region, and there is recognition that cancer cases or cancer risk factors are a major or increasing problem, and systematic organized action is required;

- the available cancer control plan is outdated in relation to the present evidence on cancer control (for example, the plan is 10 or more years old and has not been updated);

- the implemented plan is not achieving the expected outcomes, is unrealistic or limited in scope, is inefficient or inequitable, or unsatisfactory to different stakeholders;

- the available plan is reasonable, but an opportunity has arisen for a more comprehensive and effective plan – for example, there is a prospect of health sector reform in the country.

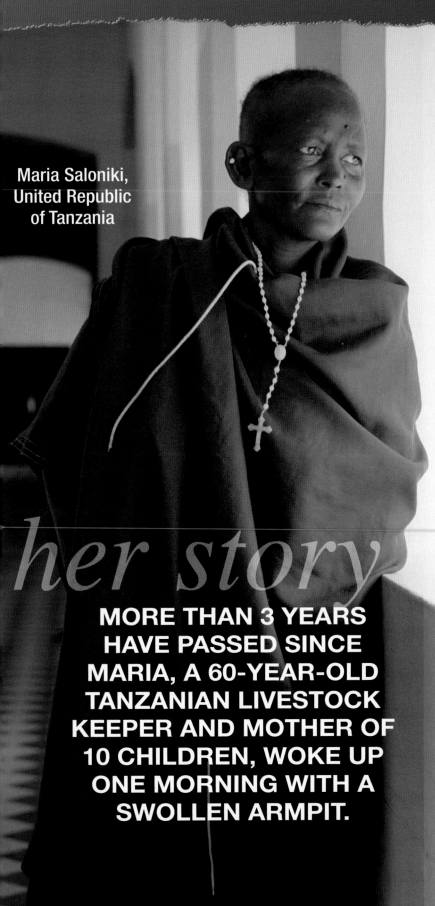

Maria Saloniki,
United Republic
of Tanzania

her story

**MORE THAN 3 YEARS
HAVE PASSED SINCE
MARIA, A 60-YEAR-OLD
TANZANIAN LIVESTOCK
KEEPER AND MOTHER OF
10 CHILDREN, WOKE UP
ONE MORNING WITH A
SWOLLEN ARMPIT.**

Maria can hardly remember how many times she went to the local traditional healer, how many doctors in clinics and dispensaries she consulted in between two hospitalizations, how many words she used to describe her pain, how many friends she turned to for advice. Maria waited more than 3 years to discover she had breast cancer – the disease was diagnosed at a very late stage with little chance of being cured.

Sadly, Maria's story is common in the understaffed and poorly equipped hospital ward she shares with 30 other cancer patients in Dar es Salaam Ocean Road Cancer Institute, the only cancer hospital in the country. Maria is one of around 24 000 cancer patients who are diagnosed with advanced cancer every year in the United Republic of Tanzania. She is also one of 2 400 cancer patients who are fortunate enough ever to reach the Ocean Road Cancer Institute.

The government recognizes that cancer is a public health problem. A national cancer control plan was endorsed by the Ministry of Health in 1997 and many steps have since been taken to improve the situation. However, the late stage at presentation does not seem to have changed much over the past 25 years. This has led policy-makers to identify past mistakes and search for new approaches.

The United Republic of Tanzania now has a unique opportunity to build on past experience and reformulate its plan of action to make it more effective. As suggested in this WHO guide, the country can consider the gradual implementation of prevention of common avoidable risk factors, the early diagnosis and treatment of a few – but frequent – cancers, and the provision of palliative care.

Source: Ngoma TA. *Report on Cancer Control Programme in Tanzania*, WHO participative workshop, 4–8 December 2000, Geneva. Additional information provided by T. Ngoma, Executive Director, Ocean Road Cancer Institute.

IF A PLAN IS NEEDED, WHO CAN ADVOCATE FOR IT?

If a new or updated cancer control plan is needed, who can champion the need for change?

Change is unlikely to occur in the absence of external stimuli. National and international organizations can act as triggers for change by influencing decision-makers in countries. Credible international organizations, such as WHO and the International Union Against Cancer (UICC), have the potential to encourage decision-makers to recognize the need for a cancer control plan in their countries.

To trigger change in a country or region, leaders with decision-making authority need to be identified and urged to take action. In the case of Chile, for example, WHO's offer to support the development of a demonstration project prompted the Chilean Minister of Health to appoint a national cancer control coordinator and council, and to develop a plan to be implemented in a stepwise manner.

Decision-makers should be reassured that a cancer control plan will not create a costly vertical programme, but can be integrated with other related programmes, which will make better use of available resources.

HOW TO DRAW UP A STRATEGIC PLAN

If national leaders decide to create a new or updated cancer control plan and if this effort survives any opposition, then the cancer control planning process can start. The planning process can be schematized as a systemic model with input, process, output, feedback and outcome, embedded in an environment (Figure 1).

It is essential to gear the planning process towards producing a cancer control plan that can be successfully implemented. A plan that is produced but not implemented within a reasonable time is a failure.

The benefits of planning are twofold: firstly, a plan is produced, and secondly, the participants in the planning process acquire knowledge and collaborative experience that will support the successful implementation of the new plan.

The planning process comprises three basic steps, providing answers, based on best evidence, to key questions:

PLANNING STEP 1:
    Where are we now?

PLANNING STEP 2:
    Where do we want to be?

PLANNING STEP 3:
    How will we get there?
    Step 3 includes two further questions:
    How will we know if we get there or not?
    How will we track progress?

Planning is an iterative cyclical process; the plan is refined through each iterative cycle. Thus, the planning and implementation steps may overlap, and it may be necessary to repeat the sequence of planning steps. For example, the priorities identified in planning step 2 may include the reorganization of cervical cancer screening in a specific target area. It may then be necessary to return to planning step 1 and do a more in-depth assessment of the services in the selected area to be able to implement the best solutions.

In the current information society, where changes occur increasingly fast, it is impossible to anticipate all possible scenarios. The plan will need the flexibility to face the unexpected and react to unplanned contingencies. The plan should also be updated regularly to make adjustments for new knowledge, new technology and customer wishes.

Figure 1. Cancer control planning process

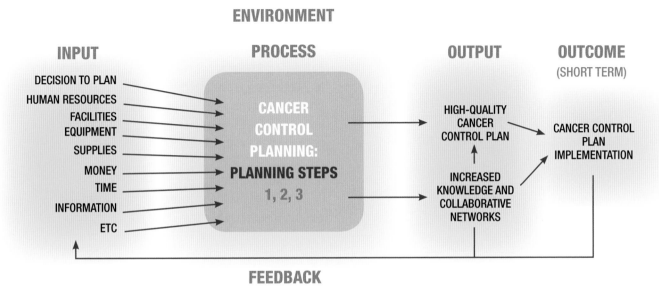

CANADA

Example of a "bottom-up" planning process

The Canadian Strategy for Cancer Control is an example of a "bottom-up" cancer control planning process with a high level of collaborative planning, within the context of a federal government.

Planning reports were produced during the course of a year of discussion, and involving consultation with over 250 cancer survivors, as well as medical and allied health professionals.

The planning process was guided by a steering committee consisting of senior executives of the Canadian Association of Provincial Cancer Agencies, the Canadian Cancer Society, the National Cancer Institute of Canada and Health Canada. It was characterized by consultation, multi-jurisdictional participation, survivor perspective and timeliness.

The process was driven by small and efficient working groups. These groups consulted broadly in developing their reports, which included as attachments written feedback submissions from stakeholders. An "integration group" consisting of representatives of national health organizations, oncology-related professional bodies, cancer survivors and the working group chairpersons, oversaw the working groups' progress and scope, and assisted in identifying gaps, integrating areas of common concern and developing the overall strategic vision.

A consultation conference was held to obtain focused input, critical comment and consensus rankings of priority actions for implementation. Participation was sought from health ministries (federal, provincial and territorial), cancer treatment centres, community cancer providers, caregivers, patients and the public to ensure that the views of both policy-makers, implementers and clients/patients were taken into account.

Source: *Canadian Strategy for Cancer Control* (http://cancercontrol. org/home_cscc.html, accessed 15 May 2006). Additional information provided by S. Sutcliffe, Chair of the Governing Council, Canadian Strategy for Cancer Control.

A good plan should be accessible and should include:

- involvement of all stakeholders,
- presentation of data on disease burden and existing control efforts,
- setting goals and objectives,
- selecting populations and strategies for intervention,
- integration of strategies with other programmes and in implementing the plan,
- resources for the implementation of the plan,
- monitoring and evaluation.

These are the components used by the State Plan Index to evaluate the quality of a written plan. The State Plan Index was developed by the United States Centers for Disease Control and Prevention (Butterfoss and Dunĕt, 2005; Dunĕt et al., 2005). It has been applied to obesity control.

Further information can be obtained at
http://www.cdc.gov/pcd/issues/2005/apr/04_0089.htm
http://www.cdc.gov/pcd/issues/2005/apr/04_0090.htm

WHO WILL DEVELOP THE CANCER CONTROL PLAN?

Who should participate in the cancer control planning process, in what ways, and during which phases?

The answer to this question will be related to a country's particular context. Several aspects, such as human resources training, and social, cultural, political, economic and technological factors could influence the selection of participants and how they participate in the cancer control planning process.

In general, "bottom-up" planning processes are preferable, as they tend to ensure that those who will put the plan into effect are involved from the beginning (see example of Canada).

Bottom-up planning may not always be possible, especially if it is contrary to the existing culture of the government, or if the only way to ensure that new resources are available is to give the government ownership of the plan. However, even in a "top-down" process a broad participatory approach is possible (see example of China).

Developing the plan involves the following stages: preparation, drafting, refinement, review, communication and marketing, budgeting and activation. These stages are shown in Table 1, with their corresponding outcomes (products) and stakeholder involvement (who is going to participate).

Another useful planning model that could be adapted to different socioeconomic contexts is known as the Building Blocks of Comprehensive Cancer Control Planning, developed in the United States by the Centers for Disease Control and Prevention (CDC) and its partners primarily to help states develop comprehensive cancer control plans (CDC, 2002).

The CDC model (see Table 2) presents specific activities to be undertaken in a loosely defined order. The first four building blocks (*enhance infrastructure, mobilize support, use data and research, build partnerships*) lay the groundwork for planning and provide a strong foundation for the entire process. The activities for the sixth building block (*conduct evaluation*) may begin very early on the process and will certainly continue throughout the implementation phases of the plan.

The fifth building block (*assess and address the cancer burden*) describes what must be done to write a plan that can be implemented and evaluated. However, if conducted prematurely or without support from the other five building blocks, the activities of this building block may well result in a plan that is neither implemented nor evaluated.

CHINA

Example of a "top-down" planning process

An example of a "top-down" cancer control planning process is provided by the Programme of Cancer Prevention and Control in China (2004–2010) initiated in 2002 and launched in 2003. China is a lower middle-income country, with a centralized government structure. Cancer represents 20% of all deaths and is, at present, the leading cause of death in urban populations. Traditionally there has been excessive reliance on treatment-oriented approaches, neglecting prevention strategies.

Alarmed by rising cancer trends, the department for disease control of the Ministry of Health initiated the planning process. A core team was in charge of developing the plan in close coordination with the prevention and control of other diseases. The major difficulty during the planning phase was to agree on the objectives and priorities of the plan. Finally, the most relevant and feasible ones were selected. In June 2003, the plan was published on the web for comments from the public. Meanwhile suggestions were collected from more than 60 experts nationwide via mail. In August 2003, the final draft was approved at a symposium that brought together relevant leaders of the Ministry of Health and other experts.

The priorities of the plan include: prevention (e.g. tobacco control, hepatitis B vaccination, control of occupational risk factors); early detection and treatment of major cancer types (uterine, cervix, breast, stomach, liver, nasopharynx, colon and rectum); rehabilitation and palliative care; and expansion of cancer registries. The biggest problem encountered in implementation is insufficient funding to carry out the biennial action plan, which mainly focuses on early detection and a public education campaign. However, there are ongoing efforts to identify further funding to support the activities.

Source: *Programme of cancer control and prevention in China, 2004–2010* (http://www.chinacancernet.org.cn/links/english.html, accessed 18 May 2006). Additional information provided by L. Kong, Deputy Director General, Disease Control Department, Ministry of Health.

Table 1. Stages in the development of a cancer control plan, their products, and potential participants

Stage	Product	Who is going to participate
Preparation	o Decide on organizational structure o Initial planning proposal o Mapping of available resources	o Small action group

Drafting	o Draft of cancer control plan
	    Planning step 1: Where are we now?
	    i.e. assessment of: cancer burden,
	    cancer control and context
	    Planning step 2: Where do we want to be?
	    i.e. identify: goals and objectives,
	    target populations, priorities
	    Planning step 3: How do we get there?
	    Action plan
	    How will we know if we get there?
	    How will we track progress?
		o Executive group
		o Planning workgroup
		o Cancer council
		o Specific task groups
		o Facilitators
		o Consultants

Refinement	o Draft with incorporated feedback	o Large reference group
Review	o Final cancer control plan	o External expert group or consultants o Executive group o Planning workgroup
Communication and marketing	o Cancer control plan disseminated o Public opinion and governmental leaders awareness	o Executive group o Specific task group
Budgeting	o Realistic pricing of the cost of initiating and maintaining the plan	o Executive group o Financial advisors
Activation	o Adoption/endorsement by the relevant national authorities	o Government (ministry of health)

Table 2. Contributions of the building blocks to the comprehensive cancer control process

Building block	Contributions
1. Enhance infrastructure	o Developing or enhancing infrastructure for planning helps initiate comprehensive cancer control, keeps it on track, and helps the process to progress.
2. Mobilize support	o Support must be mobilized both to permit initiation of the planning process and to sustain implementation and institutionalization.
3. Use data and research	o Data and research must be used to set priorities and to develop strategies to ensure that decisions are based on evidence and are defensible.
4. Build partnerships	o Partnerships must be built to ensure broad buy-in and support for both planning and implementation.
5. Assess and address the cancer burden	o This is the cornerstone of the comprehensive cancer control process supported by the other five building blocks. The cancer burden is assessed and then addressed through a broad-based partnership that enhances infrastructure, mobilizes support, uses data and research, and conducts evaluation.
6. Conduct evaluation	o Evaluation must be conducted both to monitor outcomes and to ensure continuous improvement of the process.

Source: CDC, 2002.

THE ROLE OF STAKEHOLDERS

A stakeholder is someone who has an interest in an organization or programme. Stakeholders either affect, or are affected by, the organization or programme. In the context of cancer control planning, a stakeholder has a potential to invest in the planning process.

Stakeholder analysis can be used to identify appropriate stakeholder participation. Examples of stakeholder analysis templates are:

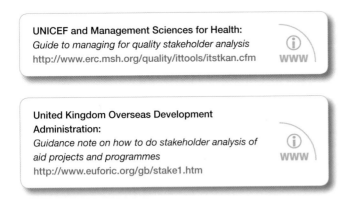

UNICEF and Management Sciences for Health:
Guide to managing for quality stakeholder analysis
http://www.erc.msh.org/quality/ittools/itstkan.cfm
WWW

United Kingdom Overseas Development Administration:
Guidance note on how to do stakeholder analysis of aid projects and programmes
http://www.euforic.org/gb/stake1.htm
WWW

If a cancer control plan is comprehensive and assuming there is a real intention to implement it, all the key current and potential stakeholders should be invited, early on, to participate in the planning process. Early involvement increases the likelihood that stakeholders will develop a sense of ownership of the plan and a commitment to making it succeed. Each partner brings his or her knowledge assets, collaborative networks and possibly other resources to the cancer control plan.

INTERACTING AND COMMUNICATING

Participants in the planning process need to interact and communicate freely. Attributes essential for collaborative work include: flexibility, open-mindedness, tolerance, acceptance of changes in authority and status, and willingness to face a challenge.

BUDGETING

To complete the cancer control planning process, there has to be a budget costing out the resources needed to implement and maintain the plan. The budget should be realistic, i.e. compatible with the resources that are likely to be made available through both government action and nongovernmental support.

PLANNING STEP 1
Where are we now?

The first step in cancer control planning is to assess the present status of the cancer problem and the cancer control activities or programmes. Because assessment of the cancer problem and the cancer control plan and programme is a complex undertaking, it is important to determine what is relevant and feasible to assess, and how to assess it.

In any effective cancer control plan, cancer control priorities and programmes are driven by available data on the cancer needs in the general population and the groups particularly at risk. Such a plan makes it possible to direct available resources or new investments to respond to unmet needs in an effective and efficient way, reducing inequalities and improving well-being.

ASSESS THE CANCER PROBLEM

Table 3 shows what to assess in relation to the needs of the general population and the groups exposed to specific risks.

Table 3. **The cancer problem: what to assess**

Population group		What to assess[a]
General population		o The social, economic and cultural context influencing the cancer problem o Demographic data o Number of healthy persons (without cancer risk factors) o Cancer and cancer risk factor awareness in the population
Population exposed to cancer risks	Tobacco	o Number of tobacco users, and tobacco use prevalence and trends o Age and gender disparities in tobacco use
	Other relevant risks	o Number, prevalence and trends for other relevant cancer risk factors, including those in the workplace and environment
Population with a new cancer	Early cancer	o Incidence of cancers amenable to early detection (e.g. cervical, breast) o Cancer stage at diagnosis o Early detection cancer awareness o Age and gender disparities in incidence, mortality, and survival of cancers amenable to early detection
	Other cancers	o Incidence of other treatable cancers o Frequency of non-curable cancers o Cancer stage at diagnosis o Cancer awareness o Prevalence of pain and other symptoms
Cancer survivor population		o Number and prevalence of cancer survivors o Cancer survival rate o Frequency of complications post-treatment or cancer-related sequelae o Number of secondary cancers o Cancer awareness o Quality of life o Psychosocial and financial needs
Cancer deaths		o Numbers of cancer deaths and mortality rates

[a]Broken down, if possible by sex, age, ethnic group, socioeconomic group and cancer site.

Basic measures of the burden of disease are the numbers of deaths, new diagnoses (incidence), people living with the disease (prevalence) and their probability of surviving the disease, and people living with terminal cancer.

The optimal resources for determining the cancer burden are:
- well organized population-based cancer registries that provide data on incidence and survival;
- good quality mortality statistics (may suffice in the absence of cancer registries).

The International Agency for Research on Cancer (IARC) is the WHO agency responsible for facilitating the establishment of cancer registries in many countries (Jensen et al., 1991; Armstrong, 1992). The International Association of Cancer Registries is another important resource in this field. National statistics are collated and made available by WHO, but coverage and completeness are uneven across countries, ranging from 100% of the population in some wealthy countries to less than 10% in Africa.

In the absence of population-based cancer registries and mortality statistics, estimates of incidence, mortality and prevalence can be derived from the relative frequency of different types of cancer (by age and sex) in any available case series. These may be patients attending one or more hospitals, for example, and it is possible that there may even be a hospital-based cancer registry from which details of these cases can be obtained.

However, the patients who attend a particular hospital are unlikely to represent a random sample of cases in the population where the hospital is situated. Cancer hospitals, for instance, will have specialized oncology services, and tend to attract patients with cancers that benefit from such treatments from a wide area, while patients with cancers that are more or less incurable (e.g. liver, lung, pancreas) will receive palliative care (if any) in local hospitals, or not be admitted at all.

Data can be obtained from the following sources, but it is important to use judgement as to how representative the information derived in this way is likely to be:
- *Hospital statistics* available from health departments are compiled for administrative purposes, and will generally refer to admissions (or discharges) rather than to cases, so that cancers requiring multiple episodes of care will be counted many times.
- *Pathology departments* often maintain case registers, so the profile of cancers diagnosed in the laboratory can be obtained; these series tend to be biased towards cancers that are readily diagnosed by biopsy, and exclude those diagnosed by other means (e.g. X-ray, ultrasound).
- *IARC* has prepared estimates of the cancer profile (incidence, mortality, prevalence) for all national populations (http://www-dep.iarc.fr/globocan/database.htm) and where neither mortality nor cancer registry data were available, it has used a variety of case series data to prepare the estimates (Ferlay et al., 2004).

> Estimates of cancer death rates for all WHO Member States are available and can be accessed at
> http://infobase.who.int
> Comparable cause of death estimates for countries are available from WHO at
> http://www.who.int/entity/healthinfo/statistics/gbdincomelevelmortality2002.xls
>
> ⓘ WWW

Where reliable population-based cancer incidence data do exist, analysis of cancer incidence and mortality data within smaller geographic units can help cancer control planners to make more informed decisions about resource allocation for screening and treatment.

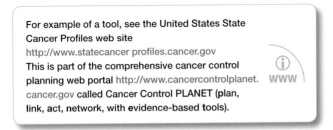

> For example of a tool, see the United States State Cancer Profiles web site
> http://www.statecancer profiles.cancer.gov
> This is part of the comprehensive cancer control planning web portal http://www.cancercontrolplanet.cancer.gov called Cancer Control PLANET (plan, link, act, network, with evidence-based tools).
>
> ⓘ WWW

It is important to compare the cancer burden, trends and projections with those for other diseases as part of the process of defining priorities. Cancer deaths represent about a quarter of total mortality in the high-income countries of the world where life expectancy is highest.

In low-income countries where life expectancy is lower, the number of cancer deaths appears to be lower. However, the increasing life expectancy in many of these countries along with an increase in exposure to cancer risk factors will eventually lead to a higher number of cancer deaths than is seen at present.

Identifying and understanding the full range of needs (i.e. physical, psychosocial, spiritual, financial) of persons exposed to risk factors, as well as those of cancer patients, their family members, their caregivers and survivors, is an important aspect of planning the services that should be made available or accessible to meet those needs. A variety of approaches can be used to identify unmet needs or degree of satisfaction of these groups.

> Further details are provided on the WHO cancer web site http://www.who.int/cancer
>
> ⓘ WWW

ASSESS THE EXISTING CANCER CONTROL PLAN AND ONGOING ACTIVITIES

Table 4 shows what to assess regarding the existing cancer control plan and ongoing activities.

Table 4. The cancer control plan and activities: what to assess

	What to assess
Cancer control plan	○ Endorsement of the plan and scope (national/provincial) ○ Timeliness (updated/outdated) ○ Accessibility to the written plan ○ Stakeholder involvement in plan development ○ Inclusion of critical sections of the plan (assessments, goals and objectives, strategies, timetable, responsible persons, resources, monitoring and evaluation) ○ Comprehensiveness and priorities (objectives and actions related to prevention, early detection, treatment, palliative care) ○ Integration with chronic disease plan and other related activities ○ Utility of the plan (used to guide programme implementation)
Ongoing cancer control activities/services and results	○ Number and type of programmes and related services offered for prevention early detection, diagnosis and treatment, palliative care ○ Coverage of ongoing activities ○ Quality of ongoing activities ○ Integration of ongoing activities with those for noncommunicable diseases and other related problems ○ Evaluation of outcomes, outputs and process indicators and trends
Resources of ongoing cancer control activities/ services	○ Information systems (e.g. cancer registries, surveillance of risk factors) ○ Protocols, guidelines, manuals, educational material etc. ○ Physical resources (infrastructure, technologies, medications) ○ Human resources (leaders, councils, committees, health-care networks, health-care providers, partners, traditional healers) ○ Financial resources ○ Regulations and legislation
The context	○ SWOT analysis: **s**trengths, **w**eaknesses, **o**pportunities and **t**hreats concerning cancer control performance

ASSESSING THE PLAN

In order to assess the cancer control plan, it is important to ask the following questions:

WHO IS ENDORSING THE PLAN AND WHAT IS THE SCOPE OF THE PLAN?

- Is the government endorsing the plan?
- Is the plan a countrywide plan or a collection of individual state or provincial plans, or is the plan limited to only one area of the country?

IS THE PLAN TIMELY?

- When was the plan developed? Is it outdated?
- Were any deadlines and responsible persons specified for the implementation of the plan?

IS THE WRITTEN PLAN ACCESSIBLE?

- Is it easily accessible in hard copies?
- Is it available on the Internet? In which languages?

HOW ARE STAKEHOLDERS INVOLVED IN THE PLAN?

Partnerships enhance the effectiveness of programmes and are most effective when they include stakeholders from different disciplines and sectors.

> See tool on assessing partnerships, available at
> http://www.who.int/cancer
>
> WWW

ASSESS STAKEHOLDER INVOLVEMENT

- Who are the partners currently involved in programme planning and implementation? Do the partners represent the diversity of stakeholder input needed? (For example, do they represent interests that are compatible with the goals of the programme?)
- What is each partner's level of engagement in the implementation of programmes of an existing cancer plan?
- Are the partners willing and ready to work together to harmonize their tasks and activities with one another in order to achieve the desired outcomes?

DOES THE PLAN INCLUDE ALL THE RELEVANT INFORMATION?

- Does the plan include a description of the cancer problem, including available data?
- Does the plan include goals, objectives, strategies (actions), resources, timetable, responsible persons to address the cancer burden, as well as monitoring and evaluation?

IS THE PLAN COMPREHENSIVE AND INTEGRATED?

- ▣ Depending on the resource level of the country, is the plan limited to one type of cancer only or focused only on one end of the cancer control continuum, when it should be broader and more comprehensive?
- ▣ Are the activities of the plan integrated with those of other related problems?

HOW USEFUL IS THE PLAN?

- ▣ Is the cancer plan a document that is used to guide programme efforts of a variety of stakeholders or is it a document that sits on the shelf and is never used?
- ▣ Has the plan ever been evaluated, and if so, how many times and when?
- ▣ What is the status of the current leadership responsible for moving cancer plan implementation forward?

ASSESSING THE PROGRAMMES OR ACTIVITIES

In assessing current cancer control programmes or activities, the focus should be on the gap between *what is needed* to address the cancer problem, and what is *currently* available.

Ask the following questions to begin to assess existing cancer programmes:

- ▣ *What programmes and related services are being offered?*
  These include direct medical service programmes as well as other support services needed to ensure high quality programmes, such as cancer registries and surveillance activities.

- ▣ *How many people and what percentage of the population are covered by the programmes?*
  This question is best answered in the context of the intended goal of the programme. For example, it may be that a cervical cancer screening programme targets only those attending maternal and child health services, and therefore does not cover the older members of the population who are most at risk of developing cervical cancer.

- ▣ *What is the quality of the programmes?*
  For each programme, it is important to ask if measures of service delivery quality have been established and monitored. If quality is assessed or could be assessed, what information is there about the adequacy of the programme in terms of meeting standards of care or the intended goals of the programme?

- ▣ *How are programmes integrated with each other and with other health programmes?*
  Health programmes that deal with cancer-related issues include: chronic disease prevention, reproductive health, occupational and environmental health, immunization for hepatitis B and HIV/AIDS. Integration of these programmes with cancer control programmes makes the best use of available resources.

- *What are the existing resources associated with these programmes?*
  Resources are listed in Table 4. Account should also be taken of the resources offered by nongovernmental organizations, for example, the number and distribution of physicians, nurses and other medical professionals in such organizations who can provide services. In some countries, it is important to consider traditional healers who, if adequately trained, can contribute to educating the community and providing supportive care.

WHAT IS THE SOCIAL AND POLITICAL CONTEXT IN WHICH PLANS AND PROGRAMMES ARE DEVELOPED?

The development of comprehensive cancer control plans and programmes requires a thorough understanding of the context. One way to assess the situation is to analyse the perceived **s**trengths, **w**eaknesses, **o**pportunities and **t**hreats (**SWOT**) associated with the existing plan and its implementation.

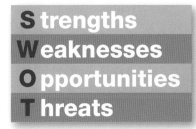

Strengths
Weaknesses
Opportunities
Threats

During the course of the **SWOT** analysis, the following questions should be answered:

- *What are the strengths and weaknesses associated with plan implementation?* These are factors affected by internal forces, such as involvement of stakeholders, political support, leadership, partner commitment to implementation, resources available to implement the plan, and evaluation efforts associated with plan implementation.

- *What are the opportunities and threats associated with plan implementation?* These are factors affected by external forces, such as a change in government leaders, the economic situation within the country, the existence of other disease priorities unrelated to cancer, and the forces underlying cancer risk or protective factors.

There are social and economic influences at work, within and among nations, that support and sustain the adoption of cancer risk-factor behaviours both intentionally and unintentionally. Perhaps the worst example of intentional support for the adoption and maintenance of a known cancer risk-factor behaviour is provided by the multinational tobacco industry (Anonymous, 2002; IARC, 2004).

Examples of unintentional promotion of cancer risk factors include industries that contribute significant concentrations of carcinogenic pollutants to the environment. Similarly, governments often fail to consider opportunities for physical activity when drawing up policies for community development, transport and the work environment. As comprehensive cancer control plans are developed, a thorough understanding of these societal and economic forces is necessary. Comprehensive cancer control programmes should address the legitimate role of community and government to regulate pro-cancer practices and adopt policies that promote health and reduce exposure to cancer risk factors (National Cancer Institute, 2000).

Table 5. Self-assessment by countries

	Core	Expanded	Desirable
Main goals of the assessment	○ To provide an overview of the extent of the cancer problem and existence and quality of the plan ○ To assess qualitatively the core elements of cancer control performance ○ To share experiences as part of the WHO web-based community	○ To assess the extent of the problem, and the quality of the current plan ○ To assess qualitatively and quantitatively some relevant elements of cancer control performance	○ To assess the social and economic context and its relationship to the cancer problem ○ To assess the extent of the problem, and the quality of the current plan ○ To assess qualitatively and quantitatively all relevant elements of cancer control performance
Primary audience	○ National and international public health community	○ National public health community	○ National public health community
Expected country coverage	○ All countries	○ Majority of countries having cancer control activities	○ Primarily countries with a well established cancer control programme
Information to be collected on the cancer burden	○ Cancer awareness in key population subgroups ○ Overall cancer incidence, and mortality and trends ○ Incidence and mortality of major avoidable, early detectable and treatable cancer types ○ Percentage of cancers diagnosed at advanced stages ○ Number of tobacco users and prevalence of tobacco use ○ Prevalence of other relevant risk factors including those related to the workplace and the environment	○ Trends in incidence and mortality of major avoidable, early detectable and treatable cancer types ○ Stage distribution of major cancer types ○ Age and gender disparities for major cancer types and cancer risk factors ○ Prevalence of pain and other frequent symptoms ○ Psychosocial and financial needs of cancer patients and their families	○ Relevant information on the socioeconomic context ○ Trends in incidence and mortality of all avoidable, early detectable and treatable cancer types ○ Trends in stage distribution ○ Number and prevalence of cancer survivors ○ Survival rates of major cancer types ○ Frequency of complications post-treatment
Information to be collected on the cancer programme	○ Simple qualitative assessment (i.e. requiring NO, YES or intermediate answers for the items listed in Table 4)	○ Quantitative information relating to ongoing cancer services and their results	○ Detailed quantitative information on outcomes, outputs and process indicators for each cancer control component
Sources of information	○ WHO/IARC statistics ○ United Nations databases ○ Ministry of health surveys	○ National statistics ○ Cancer registries ○ Population (household) surveys	○ Other national sources and interviews with opinion leaders
Information collection mechanism	○ National/local WHO team and other international organizations	○ National/local team	○ National/local team
Time frame	○ Approximately 2 months	○ Approximately 3–6 months	○ Approximately 6–8 months

SELF-ASSESSMENT BY COUNTRIES

To help countries carry out a comprehensive assessment of their cancer control situation, WHO has developed a framework for assessing population cancer needs and the existing services provided to respond to those needs. The framework follows a stepwise approach, and includes a set of self-assessment tools (core, expanded and desirable) with different levels of complexity and resource requirements.

> Self-assessment tools, which can be adapted to country circumstances, are available from the WHO web site http://www.who.int/cancer
> ⓘ WWW

Table 5 provides a summary of the different steps that should be taken within countries to assess the cancer problem and the cancer control programme.

The assessment consists of the following:

FOCUS ON PEOPLE

▣ *Consult key stakeholders* to determine the overall goals, objectives and timing of the assessment, as well as to identify a cancer control coordinator and a core assessment team.

▣ *Select a team or several teams to conduct the assessment,* and provide a clear mandate as well as a budget for support staff and advisers.

> See the WHO tool on team building at http://www.who.int/cancer
> ⓘ WWW

▣ *Define the target population,* perhaps by concentrating initially on people living in an area where cancer incidence is high (for example, an urban area rather than a rural area). If a screening programme is to be implemented, it would be wise to carry out a pilot test before expanding the programme to the rest of the country, given the cost and complexity of screening. Some cancer control interventions, such as those related to raising political awareness, may require interventions at the national level.

DATA COLLECTING

◉ *Decide on the type of assessment* (core, expanded, desirable) to be carried out (see Table 5). For example, it may be necessary to do the assessment quickly with the minimum of resources, in which case, the core assessment tool should be used. Later on, a more in-depth assessment might be carried out.

◉ *Decide on how the questions in the assessment tool can be adapted* to best meet country-specific goals and objectives.

◉ *Gather information from different sources using proper methods and techniques.* Generally, the most valuable sources of information will be national and local sources, both governmental and nongovernmental.

DATA ANALYSIS

◉ *Provide the best possible estimates, if the required information is not currently available or is very difficult to gather.* Later on, special surveys could be conducted or an information system set up to collect the information systematically.

◉ *Appraise the collected data* with regard to quality and reliability, taking into account the source of the information. Use of a standard scoring system is recommended.

> See Bandolier assessment criteria as an example at
> http://www.jr2.ox.ac.uk/bandolier/band6/b6-5.html
>
> WWW

◉ *Analyse the collected information* to identify problems in the availability and quality of services. Where there are gaps in knowledge, one priority might be to improve the quality and availability of data for future planning purposes.

REPORTING AND FOLLOW-UP

◉ *Produce a draft report.* It is advisable to circulate the draft report among stakeholders for their comments and enrichment before the final version is prepared.

◉ *Disseminate the final report widely.*

◉ *Design an action plan to bridge gaps and improve the performance of the cancer control programme.*

The self-assessment exercise will provide an answer to the question:

Where are we now?

The next planning step is to answer the question:

Where do we want to be?

PLANNING STEP 2
Where do we want to be?

The assessment (planning step 1) identifies the gaps in services, as well as in data and knowledge, with regard to the disease burden, the population at risk and the risk factors.

The next step is to consider what *could* be done, given limited resources and capacity, in order to answer the question: Where do we want to be?

DEFINE THE TARGET POPULATION

The target population of any cancer control plan depends on the goals of the plan. A comprehensive plan will cover the continuum of cancer control from prevention to palliation and target the whole population (be it of a country, region, state, province or area). A selective plan will target either a subgroup of the population or a limited component of cancer control. For example, if the plan initially focuses on palliative care, then only patients diagnosed with cancer will be the targets.

Experience gained by various countries, particularly those with limited resources and where political support is weak, shows that it is advisable to concentrate efforts on a demonstration area where a few priority initiatives are likely to be implemented successfully. These achievements can serve as entry points to attract political and financial support, allowing the programme to be expanded, at a later stage, both geographically and in scope.

IDENTIFY GAPS

Based on the assessment, the gaps can be identified (present state versus desired state), and potential corrective interventions considered.

The guiding question is: What should a person expect of the services that deliver cancer control to the population? If a cancer prevention plan is being developed, then that question is applied to the services that should be delivering best-practice cancer prevention. By comparing best practice, as reported in the world literature, with the actual services that the population is receiving, gaps in service provision become apparent.

SET OBJECTIVES

Objectives should be directly related to the gaps in cancer control that matter most for the current and future health of the population. The selection should be evidence-based and the objectives should be achievable. Objectives should be **s**pecific, **m**easurable, **a**ppropriate, **r**elevant and **t**ime bound (**SMART**). It is important to develop both outcome objectives (the expected effects on the target population) and process objectives (what needs to be done in terms of organization of activities and resources to achieve the desired outcomes).

S pecific
M easurable
A ppropriate
R elevant
T ime bound

> By placing the needs of the human being before the systems that modern man has created, we can ensure that man is indeed served by these systems rather than becoming a slave to them.

Cardinal D. *Written in the stone* (http://www.civilization.ca/cmc/architecture/tour09e.html accessed 18 May 2006).

For the plan to be effective, all the objectives need to promote a common goal. For example, early in the planning stage for the first national cancer plan in Switzerland, stakeholders set the goal: *to reduce cancer incidence and mortality and improve quality of life of patients and their families.* This goal enabled the planning team to develop objectives that focused on population needs (outcomes) and which centred the subsequent discussions on strategies and actions to match those objectives.

It is helpful to define objectives for the short term, the medium term and the long term. For example, a process measure in the *short term* could be ratification of the WHO Framework Convention on Tobacco Control. A *medium-term* outcome objective could be a 10–20% reduction in the prevalence of adult male cigarette smokers in 10 years. A corresponding *long-term* outcome objective could be a reduction in adult male lung cancer mortality by more than 10% in 20 years.

Table 6, provides examples of long- and medium-term objectives for the overall plan and its components according to the level of available resources. For each objective, there is a need to set quantifiable targets and deadlines by which to achieve them. These examples can be adapted to particular local needs, ensuring flexibility and ownership.

ASSESS FEASIBILITY OF INTERVENTIONS

The feasibility of an intervention for a given population depends on the skills and infrastructure available, the knowledge and attitudes of the target population, and the motivation of the government and cancer control providers. It is important both to assess the impact of interventions previously implemented in the target population, and to consider other interventions that have been successfully applied elsewhere.

In order to use interventions that have been effective in other populations, the characteristics of the target population should be compared with that of the other population, and the intervention adapted appropriately. For example, in cultures where important health decisions about women are usually made by men (fathers or husbands), the success of screening for breast or cervical cancer might depend on how effectively men can be educated about the benefits of that intervention.

Participation of different communities in the monitoring of activities has been one of the strengths of the international tobacco control community, interacting through the UICC Globalink web site http://www.globalink.org/ WWW

SET PRIORITIES

It is essential to set priorities, because available resources will never be able to meet all health needs. The two major determinants of priorities are the *burden of cancer* and the prevalence of cancer *risk factors*. Within the target population, the plan should aim for *equity*. The plan should deliver cancer control equitably to all members of the population at which it is aimed: the total population, a high-risk subgroup, or patients with particular cancers.

The plan must be *affordable*. Generally speaking, since cancer cannot be controlled by short-term public health strategies, it is important to ensure that there are enough resources to maintain long-term interventions, usually of indefinite duration.

In order not to waste precious resources, interventions should be *cost-effective*. A cancer control plan should include interventions that give the greatest benefit for unit cost. In low- and middle-income countries, a cancer control plan may initially be limited to prevention and palliation. The early detection of cancer on a population basis is possible only if there is an adequate primary health-care system, and enough pathologists and surgeons to follow up detected cases.

Table 6. Examples of long- and medium-term outcome objectives

	Core	Expanded	Desirable
Overall plan objectives	○ To reduce cancer incidence and mortality and improve quality of life ○ To ensure that prioritized cancer preventive and control services are provided in an equitable and sustainable way		
Prevention	○ To reduce the incidence of cancer associated with tobacco use - To reduce tobacco consumption - To reduce exposure to second-hand smoke ○ To reduce the incidence of cancer attributable to exposure to occupational and environmental carcinogens - To reduce the exposure to known carcinogens in the workplace and the environment	○ To reduce the incidence of all cancers associated with the most common avoidable risk factors - To reduce exposure to the most common avoidable risk factors	○ To reduce the incidence of rare cancers or cancers that have a genetic predisposition - To increase access to genetic testing and counselling in high-risk groups - To reduce exposure to rare avoidable risk factors
Early detection	○ To reduce mortality from cervical and breast cancers through early diagnosis - To increase the awareness of early signs and symptoms of cervical and breast cancers among patients and health-care providers, and achieve early referral to specialized clinics	○ To reduce mortality and improve survival for all cancer cases amenable to early diagnosis and cytology cervical cancer screening - To increase the awareness of early signs and symptoms of all cancer cases amenable to early diagnosis, and achieve early referral to specialized clinics - To increase the coverage of women over 35 years old with Pap smear testing every 5 years	○ To reduce mortality from breast cancer through mammography screening - To increase the coverage of women over 50 years old with mammography screening every 2 years - To ensure that all women with abnormal mammography are referred for diagnosis and treatment in specialized clinics
Diagnosis and treatment	○ To reduce mortality and improve length and quality survival of people cervical and breast cancers through prompt treatment of all cases resulting from the early diagnosis strategy - To confirm diagnosis, treat promptly, and rehabilitate as necessary all cervical and breast cancers resulting from the early diagnosis strategy	○ To reduce mortality and improve length and quality survival of people with various cancer types through prompt treatment of all cases resulting from the early diagnosis strategy - To confirm diagnosis, treat promptly, follow up and rehabilitate as necessary all cancer cases resulting from the early diagnosis strategy	○ To cure all cancers that are amenable to early detection or prolong the life significantly of disseminated cancers that have high response to treatment
Palliative care	○ To relieve advanced cancer patients from moderate/severe pain and other serious physical and psychosocial problems - To improve access to pain management and supportive care for advanced cancer patients, particularly at home and at the primary health care level	○ To relieve all advanced cancer patients from pain management and other physical and psychosocial problems - To improve access to pain management and supportive care for all advanced cancer patients at all levels of care	○ To relieve all cancer patients from suffering once they are diagnosed and improve their quality of life and that of their family members - To improve access to pain management and supportive care for all cancer patients at all levels of care

The *time frame* of the plan is important, and politicians need to be aware that few cancer control interventions can be expected to significantly alter the burden of cancer in a relatively short time. Tobacco control actions could reduce the prevalence of adult cigarette smoking in the short term, but would not immediately reduce the burden of tobacco-related cancers. A reduction in tobacco smoking among young people now would significantly reduce lung cancer rates in 40 years time.

Within 5 years, affordable improvements in the treatment of common cancers could increase survival for some patients. Within 10 years, they could start to reduce cancer mortality. Early detection and screening programmes could achieve down-staging of the targeted cancers within 5 years, and could reduce mortality within 10 years.

A plan which aims to reduce suffering from cancer in a short time frame needs to concentrate on treatment, palliation, and patient and family support. A plan which aims to reduce the total burden of cancer in a population needs to consider the whole continuum of cancer control from prevention to palliation, as well as research needs, and will have a longer timeline.

The criteria for selecting priorities will need to be discussed by the committee steering the planning process, in consultation with stakeholders. Expertly facilitated workshops can help committees to identify criteria for setting priorities (Gibson, Martin and Singer, 2004). Among the general criteria applicable to most plans (Stufflebeam, 2001), the following are particularly relevant to cancer control: political attractiveness, social values, effectiveness (in reducing the future cancer burden), and cultural context.

COST-EFFECTIVENESS ANALYSIS AS A METHOD FOR SELECTING PRIORITIES

Cost-effectiveness analysis can be used to identify not only which interventions can be implemented at a particular time for a given budget, but also those interventions that can be purchased gradually, as and when more resources become available. If resources are severely limited, it is also important to consider what proportion of the target population can be reached by the intervention. Of course, cost-effectiveness analysis also identifies cost-ineffective interventions, and so is useful in deciding which interventions not to include in the plan.

In the cancer control field, policy-makers are faced with the problem that relatively few cost-effectiveness studies have been performed, and that existing studies typically focus on a single intervention. Also, it may not be feasible to conduct cost-effectiveness analyses because the associated data and technical requirements cannot be met.

The WHO CHOICE (choosing interventions that are cost effective) project aims to meet the need for information on the cost-effectiveness of different health interventions, including cancer strategies.

Results of the project are assembled in regional databases, which policy-makers can adopt or adapt to their specific country settings (Evans, Chisholm and Tan-Torres, 2004).

Determining the priorities for a health system draws on a variety of technical, political and ethical criteria. Cost-effectiveness is never the only criterion to be considered, but it is the one that must be met most often when deciding which interventions to choose. In general, a small number of priorities, which address the major avoidable risk factors and the most prevalent cancers with cost-effective interventions, will best serve most planning purposes.

Further information on cost-effectiveness analysis for selected interventions for some cancer types can be found in the other modules of this WHO guide and on the WHO cancer web site http://www.who.int/cancer

PLANNING STEP 3
How do we get there?

What can be done with available resources? Having identified core, expanded and desirable goals, the next step is to formulate an action plan to achieve them.

A template for developing a detailed action plan is provided at http://www.who.int/cancer

The process of translating a cancer control plan into action requires competent management. It also requires a participatory approach to identify what needs to be done to reach defined goals and objectives that are feasible and sustainable.

As before, it is important to evaluate the planned actions from the perspective of those who support and will eventually implement them, and from the perspective of any opponents. Next, there is a need to identify the key person (or group) with the power to decide on the plan, and then see how that person (or group) could be activated to make the planned changes. Table 7, provides a template for this process.

Table 7. Template to identify gaps and actions to bridge them

	Level of interventions	Key actions	Who has the power to decide the key action?	How could they be activated to decide?
GAP (difference between OBSERVED and DESIRED status)	**Core** (using available resources and reorganizing the existing services)			
	Expanded (with some additional resources)			
	Desirable (with more additional resources)			

Examples of strategic changes that could improve performance with little or no increase in resources are:

- ▣ reorienting cancer screening programmes to focus on individuals at a greater risk of the disease;
- ▣ integrating cancer control more closely with other chronic disease programmes, to prevent common risk factors.

For recommendations on priorities for countries with low, middle and high levels of resources, see *National cancer control programmes: policies and managerial guidelines* (WHO, 2002).

Table 8, gives examples of priority interventions that can be implemented in a stepwise manner, starting with a low level of resources and expanding activities as more resources become available, culminating in a desired level of activities. Similarly, the interventions could be progressively implemented with increasing geographical scope or population coverage.

Tobacco control legislation and palliative care are core interventions for any setting. The organization of treatment services to manage highly curable tumours, particularly those diagnosed as a result of early detection efforts, is another priority to be implemented early, except in very low resource settings where treatment facilities are lacking.

CHILE

Example of stepwise implementation of a national cancer control programme

In 1987, with the assistance of WHO, Chile's Ministry of Health formulated a comprehensive cancer control plan and established a cancer control unit within its department of chronic diseases.

Chile adopted the basic stepwise principle of doing first what can be easily managed, and then extending the programme step by step – in Chile's case over 14 years. The initial target was the public sector, which serves 70% of the population, the majority of whom are among the less affluent and more vulnerable people of Chile.

The first implementation step comprised tobacco control activities focusing on advocacy, legislation, training and education; the reorganization of the cervical screening programme in the metropolitan area, following WHO guidelines; and the establishment of a national chemotherapy programme for selected tumours in children and adults with high potential for being cured.

The second implementation step included development and implementation of an early detection programme for breast cancer (based on awareness and physical examination) integrated with the cervical screening programme and the women's health programme; and a palliative care programme focused initially on cancer pain relief.

The third implementation step consisted of a gradual expansion of the former activities in terms of quality, quantity and scope of services to the whole country within the public system. In the past few years, all of these activities, as well as other priority cancers in the list of priority health conditions, have expanded to attain universal access to care and financial coverage. Both the public and private systems must comply with the same regulations, guidelines and protocols.

Source: Ministry of Health (2003). Plan AUGE, 2000–2010 (Universal Access System with Explicit Guarantees). Additional information provided by C. Sepúlveda, former Coordinator of the National Cancer Control Programme, Ministry of Health, Chile.

Table 8. Examples of priority interventions for each component of cancer control according to level of resources

	Core	Expanded	Desirable
Prevention	o Promote healthy behaviour and environments to reduce chronic diseases, including: - promotion of healthy diet, physical activity, safe sex, breastfeeding, and smoke-free public places - avoidance of tobacco use, abuse of alcohol and exposure to sunlight o Ratify and implement the WHO Framework Tobacco Convention o Develop regulatory and legislative measures to reduce exposure to prevalent occupational and environmental carcinogens o Integrate hepatitis B vaccination into other vaccination programmes in areas endemic for liver cancer	o Reinforce legislative measures to control tobacco use, abuse of alcohol and environmental and occupational exposure to carcinogens o Develop model community programmes for an integrated approach to prevention of chronic diseases o Develop low-cost integrated clinical preventive services for counselling on common risk factors in primary health care settings, schools and workplaces (e.g. smoking cessation and weight reduction)	o Strengthen comprehensive evidence-based health promotion and prevention programmes and ensure nationwide implementation in collaboration with other sectors o Establish routine monitoring of carcinogens if the risk of related cancers is high (e.g. ultraviolet radiation)
Early detection	o Provide early diagnosis (awareness of early signs and symptoms) of common cancers (e.g. breast and cervical) o Provide low-cost cervical cancer screening, (e.g. visual inspection with acetic acid (VIA) in demonstration projects) o Provide cytology cervical cancer screening, if facilities are available, every 10 years for at least 70% of women over 35 years old	o Provide cytology cervical cancer screening every 5 years for at least 70% of women over 35 years old o Provide services for early detection of breast cancer, and promote breast examinations by health care professionals every 1–2 years in demonstration projects or randomized trials for women over 40 years old o Develop reference training centres and quality control systems for the treatment of early detection programmes	o Provide cytology cervical cancer screening every 3 years for at least 70% of women over 25 years old o Provide mammography screening every 2 years for at least 70% of women over 50 years old o Provide colorectal cancer screening (faecal occult blood test) every 2 years for at least 70% of individuals over 50 years old
Diagnosis and treatment	o Provide diagnosis and treatment for all cancers included in an early diagnosis programme following standardized protocols o Provide diagnosis and treatment and rehabilitation as necessary for all women detected by cervical cancer screening following standardized protocols	o Provide diagnosis and treatment and rehabilitation as necessary for all disseminated cancers with high potential of being cured or significantly prolonging life (e.g. acute leukaemia in childhood, testicular seminoma), following standardized protocols o Develop/reinforce reference training centres and quality control systems for the management of priority cancers	o Reinforce the network of comprehensive cancer centres that are active for clinical training and research and give special support to the ones acting as national and international reference centres o Organize clinical trials to test new treatments that can be feasibly implemented in a variety of settings
Palliative care	o Provide pain relief and palliative care with emphasis on home-based care, following national minimum standards o Balance legislative measures to ensure access to and availability of oral morphine, and other affordable palliative care essential medications included in the WHO's essential medicines list o Develop reference centres that can provide in-service training to primary and community health caregivers	o Provide palliative care at all levels of care with emphasis on primary health care clinics and home-based care, following national protocols o Ensure availability of essential medications in both rural and urban centres o Develop reference centres that can provide undergraduate and postgraduate training o Develop curricula in both nursing and medical schools to teach palliative care both at the undergraduate and graduate levels	o Reinforce the network of palliative care services integrated with cancer and other related services o Provide support to the centres acting as national and international reference palliative care centres

RAISE THE NECESSARY RESOURCES

To make sure that the necessary human and financial resources are available to implement strategies or actions included in the plan, the following questions will need to be answered:

- What resources are currently dedicated to cancer control? How can current resources be reallocated or shared to achieve plan outcomes?
- Besides resources currently being expended, what else is needed to achieve the objectives of the plan?
- What potential sources of funding or other resources are available to meet these needs?
- How can partners work together to raise funds from government or the private sector?

A cancer control plan should be accompanied by a resource plan that outlines existing resources, needed resources and possible strategies for acquiring the needed resources from both governmental and nongovernmental sources.

WORK WITH MULTIDISCIPLINARY AND MULTISECTORAL TEAMS

Multidisciplinary and multisectoral teams are needed to implement all aspects of cancer control planning and programming. A coordinator and a board should constitute the core management team. Whenever possible, both should be appointed early in the process of establishing the cancer control plan, as they may also be in charge of coordinating the implementation.

At the local level (state, provincial, district), programme management teams and multidisciplinary health-care teams, comprising surgeons, radiotherapists, physicians (medical oncologists), cancer care nurses and social workers will have to be gradually built up as the necessary personnel are trained and become available. These teams, centred on primary health care, are the most effective means of improving cancer outcomes.

BUILD IN MONITORING AND EVALUATION

Both the development and the implementation of a cancer control plan need to be evaluated. Evaluation is a means of monitoring the planning process so that it can be improved. At the plan development level, evaluation can help answer questions about how well the planning process is working and if the goals and objectives are being met. At the plan implementation level, evaluation can show whether the strategies proposed in the plan are being implemented, and whether the anticipated outcomes are being realized.

Both outcome and process measures need to be monitored. Process evaluation is critical for laying a foundation for success in the future. Gathering feedback from key partners on their satisfaction with the planning process, then making corrections as necessary so their concerns are addressed, is an important part of building trust and credibility. The need to monitor outcome measures is evident. However, to determine whenever an intervention is likely to achieve its designed purpose, it is also necessary to monitor process measures. For example, in a cytology cervical screening programme, we need to find out whether women at high risk of cervical cancer are being screened by good quality Pap smears (process measures), and to monitor trends in incidence and mortality from cervical cancer (outcome measures), rather than simply focusing on the number of Pap smears done.

It is important to identify:
- resources and staff to conduct evaluation activities, both of plan development and implementation;
- emerging challenges, solutions and results of the planning;
- responsible persons and deadlines.

Resources and concepts related to comprehensive cancer control evaluation have been outlined by Rochester et al. (2005). WHO's *National cancer control programmes: policies and managerial guidelines* (WHO, 2002), also provides guidance on monitoring and evaluating cancer control programmes.

> Assessment tools for planning steps 2 and 3 for cancer control programmes, available in electronic format from the WHO web site at http://www. who.int/cancer provide useful guidance on how to evaluate the performance of cancer control programmes with different levels of complexity.

LAUNCH AND DISSEMINATE THE CANCER CONTROL PLAN

Once the cancer control plan is agreed upon by the stakeholders, it should be given the widest possible distribution within the country. The broader the base of understanding of the assessment results and the proposed action plan, the less difficulty there will be in implementing the necessary programme reforms. It is advisable to produce a simplified and abbreviated version of the plan that can be widely disseminated to the media and the lay public. Posting the plan on a web site will ensure accessibility. If an English version can be provided, the plan can be shared by the international community.

MOVE FROM POLICY TO IMPLEMENTATION

A plan that is developed as described in this WHO guide, and that takes account of the social and political context of the country concerned, is likely to be implemented. Effective leadership and management are essential to ensure that the right methods are applied in the right place, at the right time, with the right people to mobilize resources and move ahead.

In some countries, plans are not implemented despite political will and the support of stakeholders. This may be because the plan is too ambitious, involving costly interventions and sophisticated technologies, whereas the context is one of limited resources and competing priorities.

See example in box below. Further examples can be found at http://www.who.int/cancer

WWW

SUB-SAHARAN AFRICA

Example of constraints in moving from policy to implementation in a low-income country

In a low-income country in sub-Saharan Africa, over 8% of deaths are attributable to cancer and more than 80% of all cancer cases (estimated as 12 000 cases annually) are diagnosed at late stages. The most frequent cancer types are liver, cervical and breast cancers. There is no national health insurance policy. Cancer services take care of treatment, but these are few and very costly thus limiting access to care. Important competing problems are tuberculosis, HIV/AIDS and malaria, which elicit greater support from development agencies.

In 2002, the ministry of health of this low-income country appointed a national committee on cancer control. The following year, stimulated by the WHO country office, the chairperson of the committee, supported by a core group, drafted a cancer control plan, based on cancer control publications and plans of other countries. The ministry of health then appointed five committees (on prevention, diagnosis and treatment, palliative care, research and registry), which met in a workshop with a larger group of stakeholders to discuss and finalize the document.

The new national cancer control plan was initiated in 2003 and launched in 2004. The plan identifies the following priorities: prevention (tobacco control, alcohol control, hepatitis B vaccination); early detection through awareness of early signs and symptoms of major cancer types, and through screening for cervical cancer (using cytology), breast cancer (though breast self-examination, physical breast examination and mammography screening for high-risk groups), and prostate, bladder and testicular cancers (using clinical examination); diagnosis, treatment and rehabilitation (by reinforcing infrastructure and capacity-building for case management); and palliative care.

Cancer control is included in the health sector strategy of the national health development programme. A 5-year action plan (2006–2010) includes activities to increase or reinforce hospital-based infrastructure and build capacity, from prevention to end-of-life care.

The action plan was approved by the ministry of health. But in the 2 years since its launch, few activities have been implemented. Why? Perhaps because the plan is too ambitious, including interventions that may not be cost-effective or affordable, such as mammography screening for high-risk women, prostate screening and bone marrow transplants.

Nevertheless, the country now has an excellent opportunity to improve its cancer control plan by initially focusing efforts on a few feasible and sustainable priorities that could be implemented gradually.

In contrast, Viet Nam initiated action on cancer prevention and control in 2002, which focused in the first instance on a few priority areas. Although this action was limited in scope because of budgetary constraints, it provided a solid basis for progressing to a broader plan, which will soon be launched by the government.

VIET NAM

Example of comprehensive cancer control planning in a low-income country despite limited resources

Viet Nam is a low-income country in Asia. Chronic diseases represented 47% of the total mortality in 2002, with 8.2% attributable to cancer. The incidence is approximately 80 000 cases a year, the majority being diagnosed in very late stages.

In recent years, Viet Nam has made great efforts in cancer control despite limited resources, including the establishment of a network of cancer control centres and cancer registries in six representative areas. A national tobacco policy was adopted in 2002 consisting of measures to restrict tobacco consumption, such as banning of tobacco advertising, smoking restrictions, taxation and labelling. In 1997, hepatitis B immunization was included in the extended immunization programme for newborns in Ho Chi Minh City and Hanoi. The media were also used to disseminate information and raise awareness about cancer. Early detection of cervical cancer using cytology and low-cost alternative methods was carried out in Hanoi and some provinces, resulting in more patients coming to hospital in earlier stage of disease than in 1990–2000. Palliative care units were created in the National Cancer Hospital in Hanoi and Cho Ray General Hospital in Ho Chi Minh City.

The major difficulties encountered have been the lack of funding, equipment, facilities and trained personnel, and barriers to morphine availability for pain relief. One of the challenges has been to change the way the community thinks about cancer, especially in rural areas.

Building on the above experiences and achievements, Viet Nam developed an updated national cancer control plan for 2006–2010, which was initiated in 2002 and will be officially launched soon. Its main objectives are the following:
• reduce the incidence of tobacco-related cancers;
• ensure HBV vaccination coverage for all newborn babies;
• reduce the mortality rate in some common cancer types though early detection and timely treatment;
• improve the quality of life of cancer patients.

The updated plan was developed with the assistance of the Ministry of Health, WHO and other organizations. Financial resources derive from the state budget, as well as from national and external organizations. The action plan comprises reinforcement of the cancer control network, including the establishment of oncology departments in general hospitals in the centres of the regions, and training of health-care providers in terminal care at the provincial and community levels. The Steering Committee of the National Cancer Control Programme is in charge of monitoring and evaluation.

Source: *National Cancer Control Plan, 2006–2010.* Additional information provided by N. Duc, Director, National Cancer Hospital.

CONCLUSION

A broad participatory process that involves key stakeholders from the beginning is central to the development and implementation of an effective cancer control plan.

In resource constrained countries, a plan is more likely to be implemented if it includes fewer, yet sustainable interventions in line with evidence-based priorities, ranging from prevention to end-of-life care, with measurable process and outcome objectives that can be monitored and evaluated if basic information systems are in place. For example, prevention strategies (such as tobacco control and hepatitis B immunization), community-based palliative care for cancer and HIV/AIDS patients, and treatment interventions linked to early diagnosis (awareness of early signs and symptoms) of a few cancer types (such as cervical and breast cancers) would be key feasible interventions.

Priority interventions should be implemented using a stepwise approach, as recommended in this WHO guide, focusing initially on what can be done with better organization of available resources in a target area where there is high potential for success. As results are successfully demonstrated, more resources can be justified and the programme can be expanded.

Cancer Control
Knowledge into Action
WHO Guide for Effective Programmes

Planning

This module on cancer control planning is intended to evolve in response to national needs and experience. WHO welcomes input from countries wishing to share their successes in cancer planning. WHO also welcomes requests from countries for information relevant to their specific needs. Evidence on the barriers to cancer control in country contexts – and the lessons learned in overcoming them – would be especially welcome (contact at http://www.who.int/cancer).

REFERENCES

- Anonymous (2002). Discoveries and disclosures in the corporate documents. *Tobacco control,* 11(Suppl. 1):1–117.

- Armstrong BK (1992). The role of the cancer registry in cancer control. *Cancer causes and control,* 3:569–579.

- Butterfoss FD, Duñet DO (2005). State Plan Index: a tool for assessing the quality of state public health plans. *Preventing chronic disease,* A15.

- CDC (2002). *Guidance for comprehensive cancer control planning.* Atlanta, GA, United States. Department of Health and Human Services, National Institute of Health.

- Duñet DO et al. (2005). Using the State Plan Index to evaluate the quality of state plans to prevent obesity and other chronic diseases. *Preventing chronic disease,* 2:A10.

- Evans D, Chisholm D, Tan-Torres T (2004). *Generalized cost-effectiveness analysis: principles and practice.* Geneva, World Health Organization.

- Ferlay J et al. (2004). *GLOBOCAN 2002. Cancer incidence, mortality and prevalence worldwide.* Lyon, International Agency for Research on Cancer (*IARC CancerBase No. 5,* version 2.0).

- Gibson JL, Martin DK, Singer PA (2004). Setting priorities in health care organizations: criteria, processes, and parameters of success. *BMC Health Services Research:* 1–8.

- IARC (2004). *Tobacco smoke and involuntary smoking.* Lyon, International Agency for Research on Cancer (IARC Monographs on the Evaluation of Carcinogenic Risks to Humans, Volume 83).

- Jensen OM et al., eds (1991). *Cancer registration principles and methods.* Lyon, International Agency for Research on Cancer (IARC Scientific Publications No. 95).

- Mintzberg H (1994). *The rise and fall of strategic planning.* New York, NY, The Free Press.

- National Cancer Institute (2000). *State and local legislative action to reduce tobacco use.* Bethesda, MD, United States Department of Health and Human Services, National Institute of Health (*Smoking and Tobacco Control Monograph No. 11,* NIH Pub. No. 004804*).*

- Rochester P et al. (2005). The evaluation of comprehensive cancer control efforts: useful techniques and unique requirements. *Cancer causes and control,* 16:69–78.

- Stufflebeam DL (2001). *Evaluation values and criteria checklist.* (http://www.wmich.edu/evalctr/checklists/values_criteria.htm, accessed 24 April 2006).

- WHO (2002). *National cancer control programmes: policies and managerial guidelines.* Geneva, World Health Organization.

- WHO (2005). *Preventing chronic diseases: a vital investment.* Geneva, World Health Organization.

ACKNOWLEDGEMENTS

WHO THANKS THE FOLLOWING EXTERNAL EXPERTS FOR REVIEWING DRAFT VERSIONS OF THE MODULE. EXPERT REVIEWERS DO NOT NECESSARILY ENDORSE THE FULL CONTENTS OF THE FINAL VERSION.

Tiiu Aareleid, Estonian Cancer Registry, North Estonian Regional Hospital's Cancer Centre, Estonia
A. M. M. Shariful Alam, National Institute of Cancer Research & Hospital, Bangladesh
Yasantha Ariyaratne, National Cancer Control Programme, Sri Lanka
Dilyara Barzani, Hawler Medical University, Ministry of Health, Kurdistan Regional Government, Iraq
Felix Bautista, Multisectoral Coalition Against Cancer, Peru
Yasmin Bhurgri, Karachi Cancer Registry & Aga Khan University Karachi, Pakistan
Barry D. Bultz, Tom Baker Cancer Centre and University of Calgary, Canada
Lidieth Carballo, Ministry of Health, Costa Rica
Arkom Cheirsilpa, National Cancer Institute, Thailand
Frances Prescilla L. Cuevas, National Center for Disease Prevention and Control, Department of Health, Philippines
Lea Derio, Ministry of Health, Chile
Ketayun A. Dinshaw, Tata Memorial Centre, India
Anderson S. Doh, Faculty of Medicine and Biomedical Sciences, Cameroon
George Gellert, International Atomic Energy Agency, Austria
Charles Gombé-Mbalawa, Faculty of Medicine, University of Brazzaville, Congo
Maisoon Juhani, Ministry of Health, Syrian Arab Republic
Elona Juozaityte, Kaunas Medical University, Lithuania

Neeta Kumar, Geneva, Switzerland
Juozas Kurtinaitis, Institute of Oncology, Vilnius University, Lithuania
Abel Limache, Multisectoral Coalition Against Cancer, Peru
M. Krishnan Nair, Regional Cancer Centre, India
Twalib A. Ngoma, Ocean Road Cancer Institute, United Republic of Tanzania
Zainal A. Omar, Ministry of Health, Malaysia
D. M. Parkin, Clinical Trials Service Unit and Epidemiological Studies Unit, England
Luis Pinillos, Multisectoral Coalition Against Cancer, Peru
Roger Pla i Farnós, Department for Coordination of Master Plans, Department of Health, Regional Government of Catalonia, Spain
Erzsébet Podmaniczky, National Institute of Oncology, Hungary
Marta Prieto, Ministry of Health, Chile
You-Lin Qiao, Chinese Academy of Medical Sciences and Peking Union Medical College, China
Mahmudur Rahman, Institute of Epidemiology, Disease Control and Research, Bangladesh
Eliezer Robinson, National Council for Oncology and Israeli Cancer Association, Israel
Miguel Ruiz, Multisectoral Coalition Against Cancer, Peru
Anne Lise Ryel, Norwegian Cancer Society, Norway
Dolores Salas Trejo, Department of Health, Regional Government of Valencia, Spain
Thida San, Yangon General Hospital, Myanmar
Luiz Antônio Santini Rodrigues da Silva, National Cancer Institute, Brazil
Kavita Sarwal, Canadian Strategy for Cancer Control, Canada
Hai-Rim Shin, National Cancer Center, Republic of Korea

Cecilia Solis-Rosas García, Ministry of Health, Peru
Eugenio Suárez, Ministry of Health, Chile
Simon Sutcliffe, British Columbia Cancer Agency, Canada
Luis Távara, Multisectoral Coalition Against Cancer, Peru
Maja Primic Žakelj, Institute of Oncology, Slovenia

THE FOLLOWING WHO STAFF ALSO REVIEWED DRAFT VERSIONS OF THE MODULES

WHO regional and country offices
Roberto Eduardo del Aguila, WHO Costa Rica Country Office
Gauden Galea, WHO Regional Office for the Western Pacific
Jerzy Leowski, WHO Regional Office for South-East Asia
Silvana Luciani, WHO Regional Office for the Americas
Cherian Varghese, WHO India Country Office

WHO headquarters
Robert Beaglehole
Rafael Bengoa
Nathalie Broutet
Serge Resnikoff
Andreas Ullrich

WHO CANCER TECHICAL GROUP
The members of the WHO Cancer Technical Group and participants in the first and second Cancer Technical Group Meetings (Geneva 7–9 June and Vancouver 27–28 October 2005) provided valuable technical guidance on the framework, development, and content of the overall publication, *Cancer control: knowledge into action*.

Baffour Awuah, Komfo Anokye Teaching Hospital, Ghana

Volker Beck, Deutsche Krebsgesellschaft e.V, Germany

Yasmin Bhurgri, Karachi Cancer Registry & Aga Khan University Karachi, Pakistan

Vladimir N. Bogatyrev, Russian Oncological Research Centre, Russian Federation

Heather Bryant, Alberta Cancer Board, Division of Population Health and Information, Canada

Robert Burton, WHO China Country Office, China

Eduardo L. Cazap, Latin-American and Caribbean Society of Medical Oncology, Argentina

Mark Clanton, National Cancer Institute, USA

Margaret Fitch, International Society of Nurses in Cancer Care and Canada, Toronto Sunnybrook Regional Cancer Centre, Canada

Kathleen Foley, Memorial Sloan-Kettering Cancer Center, USA

Leslie S. Given, Centers for Disease Control and Prevention, USA

Nabiha Gueddana, Ministry of Public Health, Tunisia

Anton G.J.M. Hanselaar, Dutch Cancer Society, the Netherlands

Christoffer Johansen, Danish Institute of Cancer Epidemiology, Danish Cancer Society, Denmark

Ian Magrath, International Network for Cancer Treatment and Research, Belgium

Anthony Miller, University of Toronto, Canada

M. Krishnan Nair, Regional Cancer Centre, India

Twalib A. Ngoma, Ocean Road Cancer Institute, United Republic of Tanzania

D. M. Parkin, Clinical Trials Service Unit and Epidemiological Studies Unit, England

Julietta Patnick, NHS Cancer Screening Programmes, England

Paola Pisani, International Agency for Research on Cancer, France

You-Lin Qiao, Cancer Institute, Chinese Academy of Medical Sciences and Peking Union Medical College, China

Eduardo Rosenblatt, International Atomic Energy Agency, Austria

Michael Rosenthal, International Atomic Energy Agency, Austria

Anne Lise Ryel, Norwegian Cancer Society, Norway

Inés Salas, University of Santiago, Chile

Hélène Sancho-Garnier, Centre Val d'Aurelle-Paul Lamarque, France

Hai-Rim Shin, National Cancer Center, Republic of Korea

José Gomes Temporão, Ministry of Health, Brazil

Other participants

Barry D. Bultz, Tom Baker Cancer Centre and University of Calgary, Canada

Jon F. Kerner, National Cancer Institute, USA

Luiz Antônio Santini Rodrigues da Silva, National Cancer Institute, Brazil

Observers

Benjamin Anderson, Breast Health Center, University of Washington School of Medicine, USA

Maria Stella de Sabata, International Union Against Cancer, Switzerland

Joe Harford, National Cancer Institute, USA

Jo Kennelly, National Cancer Institute of Canada, Canada

Luiz Figueiredo Mathias, National Cancer Institute, Brazil

Les Mery, Public Health Agency of Canada, Canada

Kavita Sarwal, Canadian Strategy for Cancer Control, Canada

Nina Solberg, Norwegian Cancer Society, Norway

Cynthia Vinson, National Cancer Institute, USA